THE TREATMENT

A SIMPLE STEP BY STEP GUIDE

FOR TREATING VERTIGO

BOBBY GIBBS

Copyright © 2016 by Bobby Gibbs

All Rights Reserved. No part of this book may be reproduced, stored in a retrieval system, or transmitted, in any form or by any means, electronic, mechanical, photocopying, recording, or otherwise, without the prior written permission of the author.

This book is presented for educational and information purposes, and to increase the public knowledge and awareness of developments in the field of vertigo and vestibular disorders. The information outlined herein should not be adopted without a consultation with your health professional.

Use of the information provided is at the sole choice and risk of the reader. You must get your physician's approval before beginning any of the exercises or techniques within this book. This information is not a prescription. Consult with your doctor or health professional for further information. Neither the author nor the publisher accept liability for readers who choose to self-prescribe.

Cover and interior design by Bobby Gibbs

ISBN: 978-1-52076-928-8

Table of Contents

Welcome	4
About Bobby Gibbs	5
Stage 1: Introduction	6
Stage 2: A Scientific View of the Vertigo Treatment guide	10
Stage 3: The Vital Steps of Training	14
Stage 4: Your Journal	19
Stage 5: Balance Tests	25
Stage 6: Breakpoint Exercise: Abdominal Breathing	49
Stage 7: Levels of Vestibular Progression	51
Stage 8: The Exercises	54
Stage 9: What Next?	94

Welcome

Hello there, and thanks for investing your time into the Vertigo Treatment guide.

My mission is to make sure that you're in good hands and that you get the most out of this guide. I have personally dedicated thousands of hours into combining and implementing the best approaches that you can take to ensure your body is at an optimal state.

Thanks to Neuroplasticity which allows us to reshape and restructure our brains, we'll be going through a journey taking you from where you are now, to a state of health and well-being.

Let us now embark upon this journey together and see what is in store for you.

About Bobby Gibbs

As a vestibular personal trainer and life coach, I have lived with vestibular neuritis and BPPV (benign paroxysimal positional vertigo) for over 3 years. During this time I have come across various health and fitness related practices, routines and remedies that have significantly improved my condition.

This brings me to the reason I decided to create Cure Vertigo Now, as I want to help others who are going through similar experiences and who may be suffering from vertigo or vestibular disorders.

The information presented here is intended to provide you with the necessary exercises to facilitate and improve vertigo or vestibular-related issues. So if you to want make some positive and dramatic changes in your health, this is the program for you.

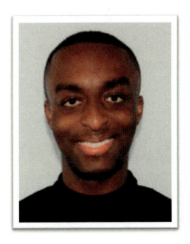

Stage 1: Introduction

What is the Vertigo Treatment guide?

The Vertigo treatment guide consists of a variety of exercises that use the concept of Neuroplasticity (the brain's ability to reprogram and remodel itself) to enhance balance and improve the vestibular system. Training and challenging the vestibular system will also train the nervous system to stop and reduce any sensations of vertigo and dizziness. In addition, these exercises have been designed to make everyday movement much more seamless and efficient.

We have ensured to make the Vertigo Treatment guide a simple step-by-step process that includes the most essential and important factors to help to reduce vertigo, dizziness, pain and inefficient movement patterns.

How does the Vertigo Treatment guide work?

The Vertigo Treatment guide is focused on improving balance, making movement graceful and stopping signs of dizziness and vertigo. This works because of 2 fundamental principles:

1.) Neural Signal Quality – Neural signals are sent all over your body thanks to your nervous system. It's vital that the quality of neural signals is good; otherwise, your body will not perform at its peak. In particular, we want to ensure that neural signals for our eyes, vestibular system and proprioceptive system are optimal to really get the most benefit for our movement and balance. To make this happen we must activate, train and challenge all 3 of these areas.

2.) Body Signal Integration – As well as having optimal neural signal quality, great body signal integration is necessary. Body signal integration is the way your brain takes in and processes the information coming in from the eyes, vestibular system and proprioceptive system. In essence, your body knows how to balance due to your brain; this means that to enhance the body's level of body signal integration, we must train and challenge our brain. All the exercises within the Vertigo Treatment guide have been put together to improve this important ability.

The Benefits

As you take part in the exercises and further improve your condition, your body will go through some amazing changes. Below are some of the benefits that we and our clients have experienced, that will take your body to a whole new level:

*Better body movement.

*Better balance.

*Enhanced spatial awareness.

*Improved body posture.

*Increased range of motion of muscles.

*Increases in strength, endurance and overall better performance at sports and day-to-day activities.

*Reduction and prevention of dizzy spells.

*Major reduction in blurred vision and better gaze fixation.

*Reduction in joint and muscle pain throughout the body.

*More confidence when walking and performing daily activities.

*Higher energy levels and reduction in fatigue.

*And more!

You may experience some of these benefits when you first start doing the exercises. Others may take a while to kick in, so PLEASE BE PATIENT!

It's also important to record your progress within your journal so that you can reflect back on your progression and see how far you've come along throughout your journey. The important thing is to ensure that you KEEP ON DOING THE EXERCISES!

Stage 2: A Scientific View of the Vertigo Treatment Guide

I know that you're probably eager to delve into the exercises provided within this guide, but we encourage you to take the time out to also go over the science behind why these profound exercises work and why they play a significant role in your training. By gaining a scientific understanding of this guide it will allow you to make unique adjustments to your own training routines and see what is truly working for you, enabling you to gain even more benefits.

The Vestibular System

In simple terms, your vestibular system is in charge of keeping you balanced and maintaining a nice upright equilibrium in relation to gravity and your surroundings. This works mainly when body and head movements are stimulated; each time you move your head, you are activating neural signals which get sent to your vestibular system, where it integrates (puts together) sensory information coming from your entire body and processes this all within the brain. This is able to happen thanks to your nervous system.

Your vestibular system does the following:

*Lets your body know where you are in regards to your surroundings and the space around you.

*Controls and plans out the best movements for you to take in order to move around as efficiently and gracefully as possible.

*Plays a part in how fast your body movements are being carried out.

*Maintains and keeps you upright in relation to gravity and your surroundings.

In addition, our 3 sensory systems also come into play.

The 3 Sensory Systems

Within our body we have our nervous system, which governs and controls how our body operates and functions. In conjunction with this, our nervous system works with our 3 sensory systems. They are as follows:

*The visual system

*The vestibular system (also known as the inner ear)

*The proprioceptive system (also known as our movement system)

These 3 sensory systems integrate and combine all the sensory information that the body receives together, where everything is processed within the brain. If one of these sensory systems isn't functioning optimally (e.g. due to injury or a disorder) then this can cause negative outcomes such as pain, dizziness, jerky eye movements, loss of balance and much more.

This is why it's essential to have great neural signal quality; it will enable you to avoid having any of these symptoms from taking place. By having great neural signal quality, it allows us to have the most efficient movement and balance, and prevents symptoms such as vertigo or loss of balance from occurring. If these issues aren't corrected, they can lead to more on going issues.

As stress builds up in the body, muscle tension, fear, lack of confidence, anxiety, fatigue and more issues can begin to manifest. No one wants to live their lives with any of these issues, which is why we can't emphasize enough how important it is that these 3 sensory systems function properly.

How Small Problems Lead to Bigger Problems

Even if there is a small problem with how your vestibular system is functioning, overall it can have a big impact on your performance and your sense of balance. For example, if you notice that moving your head to the left is a little jerky and more difficult in comparison with moving your head to the right, this can have a major influence in terms of how your overall vestibular system functions and operates. This small problem could be the reason why you may be experiencing some pain in your lower back, or the reason why you may find walking with your right leg easier in comparison with your left leg.

There's also the fact that when one is afraid that they may fall over, the instinctive reaction of the human body is to tense up; this is a survival mechanism that has been programmed into the nervous system. But if you were to continue to go through this cycle of being fearful every time you may slip or fall over, it creates more stress and tension within the body, which leads to a myriad of other problems.

This is why, as well as having good balance, it's very important that you are relaxed and breathing well at all times to avoid these negative effects. Rather than settling for you being afraid every time you take a step, this guide has been designed to transform you into someone who moves around with grace and confidence.

Stage 3: The Vital Steps of Training Balance

Alright, so we understand that to improve balance we must follow 2 main principles:

*We must improve neural signal quality.

*We must improve body signal integration.

However, as well as following these 2 main principles, there are several rules that we must also abide by in order for us to really reap the benefits. They are as follows:

We must work with our VISUAL SYSTEM – to do this we must:

*Move our head when our eyes are kept still.

*Move our eyes when our head is kept still.

*Move our eyes and head in opposite directions.

We must work with our VESTIBULAR SYSTEM (inner ear) – to do this we must:

*Rotate our head.

*Nod our head.

*Perform diagonal movements with our head.

We must work with our PROPRIOCEPTIVE SYSTEM – to do this we must:

*Train our body on a step-by-step basis by starting at lying down, then sitting, then standing on both feet, then standing with one foot in front of the other (also known as tandem standing), then standing on one foot, then walking.

*Train with the eyes open first, then advance to training with the eyes closed.

We must work to improve our body and brain integration – to do this we must:

*Use and put together all of the above exercises as walking exercises and movements.

Prerequisites

Step 1: Do The Exercises Safely!

When doing these exercises, please ensure that your environment is safe. This means that no dangerous or sharp objects are to be nearby. In addition, make sure that you have a form of support such as a wall or chair nearby. As we are training the vestibular system and working on improving your balance, it's important that you don't fall over and that you are safe and comfortable when performing the exercises.

Step 2: Speak With Your Physician Before Doing The Exercises

As an additional safety precaution, it's a good idea to consult with your physician or doctor. As we don't know the state and condition your body is currently at, these exercises may not be the most suitable course of action for you to take. So to be extra safe here, we recommend that you follow this step.

Step 3: Get The Support of Someone Close To You

These exercises can be challenging and it's always great to have someone supporting you. With that said, get someone who's close to you to do just that and encourage you as you're doing the exercises.

Step 4: Gain Feedback

This step is very important and could potentially save you from doing some of the exercises incorrectly. Wouldn't it be disappointing if you skipped this step, only to find out that for several months you had been doing the exercises wrong? Having someone to provide you feedback on the exercises is very useful as they can tell you how well you're doing the exercises and can also advise you if there is room for improvement.

If you're unable to get the support of another, then using a mirror can be invaluable for checking how well you are doing the exercises. For example, this can help to ensure that you are moving your head smoothly and not jerking it. Another measure that you can take is to record yourself with a webcam. This is a great way of monitoring and keeping track of your progress, where you can see how well you've progressed over the months.

Step 5: Do The Exercises Barefoot

To get the most benefits from the exercises it's ideal to train barefoot. When training barefoot it allows you to fully train your vestibular system and sense of balance. By wearing shoes it makes the exercises less challenging and doesn't allow you to make direct contact with the ground. You can also wear socks, but going barefoot will allow you to gain the best results from the exercises.

Step 6: Make Sure That You Relax

You need to be in a relaxed state when doing these exercises. This means that your body shouldn't be tense when performing any of the exercises and that you shouldn't be holding your breath. This will only trigger the fight-or-flight response, which is the body's way of reacting to stress or danger and is something that we do not want to encourage. In addition to this, we don't want to develop bad habits, meaning that we don't want to train your body where, for example, every time you moved your head to the right you held your breath. This is why being in a relaxed and calm state as well as breathing correctly will help to boost the effects of your training.

Step 7: How Regularly Do I Need To Do The Exercises?

As well as training the vestibular system you need to ensure that you also include periods of rest. Below is the recommendation for how you should train:

*10 minutes a day

*3-5 days per week

Remember that the above recommendation is only a guide. Even though this is the recommended training amount, it can vary from person to person. You may find that doing the exercises for only 5 minutes a day, 7 days a week is more beneficial for you. This is why it's important to record how you react and feel after doing the exercises.

> **Bonus Tip**
> We also suggest that you space out your sessions, so that you do them 2-4 times in one day. This means that you could have a 5 minute session in the morning and a 5 minute session in the evening. By spacing out your sessions it prevents you from overwhelming your brain and bringing on any signs of excessive dizziness.

Stage 4: Your Journal

Training is one thing, but we can't train without keeping track of our results. We want to ensure that you know what exercises are working best for you and which ones may be giving you no results. This is where your journal comes into play. This journal has been broken down into a 12 week process, giving you the ability to monitor how you're performing.

Keep in mind that an exercise that is good for you may not be good or effective for someone else. This is why we've included a journal for you to take note of your progression.

> **Bonus Tips**
>
> A.) We recommend that you track your results daily, even on the days that you are resting and not training. By monitoring your progress each day you are giving yourself more clarity upon how far you've progressed and can make some adjustments to your training routine. It will also help to indicate what exercises may not be working out so well for you.
>
> B.) Remember to vary the exercises that you perform each week so that your body adapts to them.

12 Week Journal

	Time Balanced For	Daily Exercise/s	Standing Position/s used	Notes
Day 1	20secs	Balance tests	Balancing on 1 leg	Found it hard to balance on 1 leg with eyes closed.
Day 2	1min	1 exercise (3mins max) & breakpoint exercise	Wide foot position	Distant gaze stabilization – Did 2 reps in all directions at a slow speed. Will increase speed with more practice.
Day 3	20secs	Balance tests	Balancing on 1 leg	Felt a little easier to balance with eyes closed.
Day 4	2mins	1 exercise (3mins max) & breakpoint exercise	Normal foot position	Close range gaze stabilization – Felt harder to do in comparison with distant gaze exercise. Did 2 reps in all directions.

Here is a short example of how you can fill in your 12 week journal.

12 Week Journal

	Time Balanced For	Daily Exercise/s	Standing Position/s Used	Notes
Day 1		Balance tests		
Day 2		1 exercise (3 mins max) & breakpoint exercise		
Day 3		Balance tests		
Day 4		1 exercise (3 mins max) & breakpoint exercise		
Day 5		Balance tests		
Day 6		1 exercise (3 mins max) & breakpoint exercise		
Day 7		Rest		
Day 8		Balance tests		
Day 9		1 exercise (3 mins max) & breakpoint exercise		
Day 10		1 exercise (3 mins max) & breakpoint exercise		
Day 11		Rest		
Day 12		1 exercise (3mins max) & breakpoint exercise		
Day 13		Balance tests		
Day 14		Rest		
Day 15		1 exercise (6 mins max) & breakpoint exercise		
Day 16		Balance tests		
Day 17		1 exercise (6 mins max) & breakpoint exercise		
Day 18		Balance tests		
Day 19		1 exercise (6 mins max) & breakpoint exercise		
Day 20		Balance tests		
Day 21		Rest		
Day 22		Balance tests		
Day 23		1 exercise (6 mins max) & breakpoint exercise		
Day 24		1 exercise (6 mins max) & breakpoint exercise		

12 Week Journal

	Time Balanced For	Daily Exercise/s	Standing Position/s Used	Notes
Day 25		Rest		
Day 26		1 exercise (6 mins max) & breakpoint exercise		
Day 27		Balance tests		
Day 28		Rest		
Day 29		1 exercise (10 mins max) & breakpoint exercise		
Day 30		Balance tests		
Day 31		1 exercise (10 mins max) & breakpoint exercise		
Day 32		Balance tests		
Day 33		1 exercise (10 mins max) & breakpoint exercise		
Day 34		Balance tests		
Day 35		Rest		
Day 36		Balance tests		
Day 37		1 exercise (10 mins max) & breakpoint exercise		
Day 38		1 exercise (10 mins max) & breakpoint exercise		
Day 39		Rest		
Day 40		1 exercise (10 mins max) & breakpoint exercise		
Day 41		Balance tests		
Day 42		Rest		
Day 43		Balance tests		
Day 44		2 exercises (10 mins max) & breakpoint exercise		
Day 45		2 exercises (10 mins max) & breakpoint exercise		
Day 46		Rest		
Day 47		2 exercises (10 mins max) & breakpoint exercise		
Day 48		Balance tests		

12 Week Journal

	Time Balanced For	Daily Exercise/s	Standing Position/s Used	Notes
Day 49		Rest		
Day 50		3 exercises (10 mins max) & breakpoint exercise		
Day 51		Balance tests		
Day 52		3 exercises (10 mins max) & breakpoint exercise		
Day 53		Balance tests		
Day 54		3 exercises (10 mins max) & breakpoint exercise		
Day 55		Balance tests		
Day 56		Rest		
Day 57		Balance tests		
Day 58		3 exercises (10 mins max) & breakpoint exercise		
Day 59		3 exercises (10 mins max) & breakpoint exercise		
Day 60		Rest		
Day 61		3 exercises (10 mins max) & breakpoint exercise		
Day 62		Balance tests		
Day 63		Rest		
Day 64		4 exercises (10 mins max) & breakpoint exercise		
Day 65		Balance tests		
Day 66		4 exercises (10 mins max) & breakpoint exercise		
Day 67		Balance tests		
Day 68		4 exercises (10 mins max) & breakpoint exercise		
Day 69		Balance tests		
Day 70		Rest		
Day 71		All exercises (10 mins max) & breakpoint exercise		
Day 72		Balance tests		

12 Week Journal

	Time Balanced For	Daily Exercise/s	Standing Position/s Used	Notes
Day 73		All exercises (10 mins max) & breakpoint exercise		
Day 74		Balance tests		
Day 75		All exercises (10 mins max) & breakpoint exercise		
Day 76		Balance tests		
Day 77		Rest		
Day 78		Balance tests		
Day 79		All exercises (10 mins max) & breakpoint exercise		
Day 80		All exercises (10 mins max) & breakpoint exercise		
Day 81		Rest		
Day 82		All exercises (10 mins max) & breakpoint exercise		
Day 83		Balance tests		
Day 84		Rest		

Stage 5: Balance Tests

The balance tests are a way of assessing and gaining instant feedback on the current state of your balance and vestibular system. They are great for seeing how far you've progressed; ensure you do them regularly.

> **Bonus Tip**
> Before beginning these balance tests, be sure that you're doing them in a safe environment. Have a chair or wall nearby to support you and prevent you from falling.

Test Out How You Feel

When doing these tests assess yourself on the following:

*Am I able to do the exercises?

*Is it easy or hard for me to perform each exercise?

*For what length of time can I do each test?

What we're aiming to achieve here is to make doing these tests as simple and easy as possible, where you're able to do them for a long length of time in succession.

Balance Test 1 – Difficulty: Easiest

Sitting with various head movements

Step 1 – Keeping head still with eyes opened

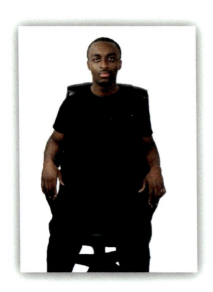

*Sit comfortably on a chair facing forward.

*With eyes open, keep the body still for 20 seconds.

*Make a note of how you feel.

Step 2 – Keeping eyes closed with head still

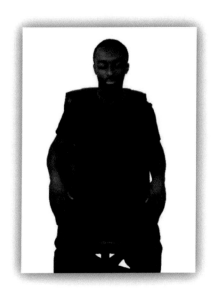

*Repeat the above step but with eyes closed.

Step 3 – Rotating head with eyes open

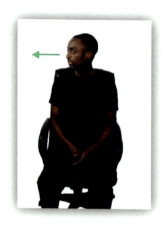 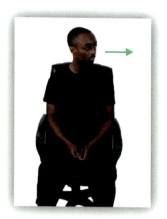

*Sit comfortably on a chair facing forward.

*Rotate your head left and right for 20 seconds.

*Make a note of how you feel.

Step 4 – Rotating head with eyes closed

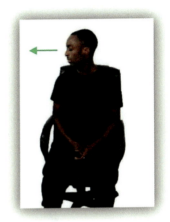 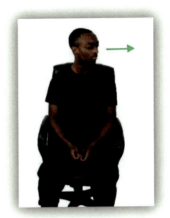

*Repeat the above step but with eyes closed.

Step 5 – Nodding head with eyes open

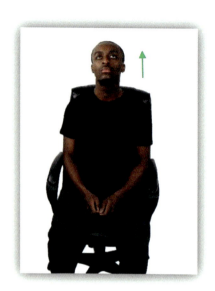

*Sit comfortably on a chair facing forward.

*Nod head upwards and downwards for 20 seconds.

*Make a note of how you feel.

Step 6 – Nodding head with eyes closed

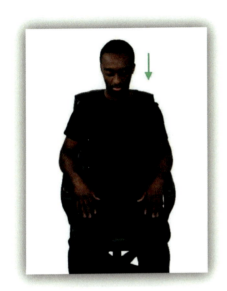

*Repeat the above step but with eyes closed.

Balance Test 2 – Difficulty: Easy

Standing normally with various head movements

Step 1 – Keeping head still with eyes open

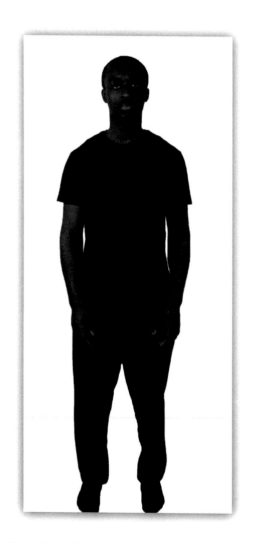

*Stand comfortably, keeping feet facing forward.

*With eyes open, keep the body still for 20 seconds.

*Make a note of how you feel.

Step 2 – Keeping eyes closed with head still

*Repeat the above step but with eyes closed.

Step 3 – Rotating head with eyes open

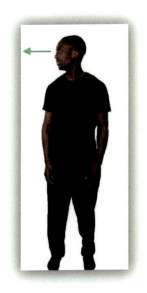 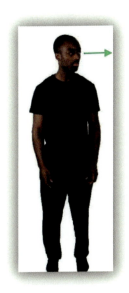

*Stand comfortably keeping feet facing forward.

*Rotate your head left and right for 20 seconds.

*Make a note of how you feel.

Step 4 – Rotating head with eyes closed

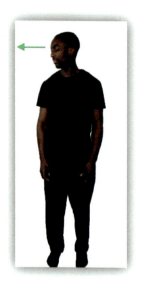 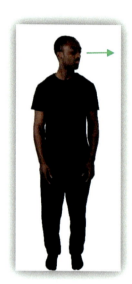

*Repeat the above step but with eyes closed.

Step 5 – Nodding head with eyes open

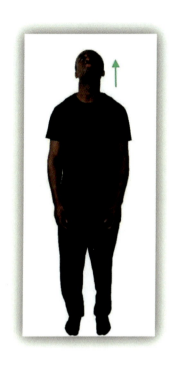

*Stand comfortably keeping feet facing forward.

*Nod head upwards and downwards for 20 seconds.

*Make a note of how you feel.

Step 6 – Nodding head with eyes closed

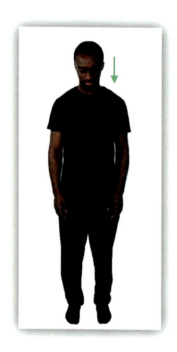

*Repeat the above step but with eyes closed.

Balance Test 3 – Difficulty: Intermediate

Narrow Standing with various head movements

Step 1 – Keeping head still with eyes open

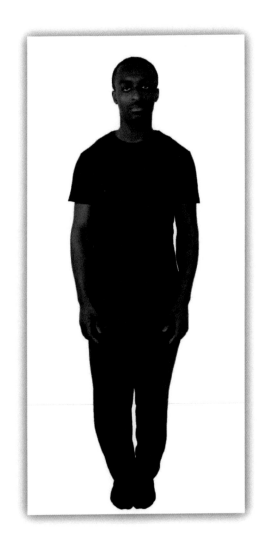

*Stand comfortably keeping feet close together, facing forward.

*With eyes open, keep the body still for 20 seconds.

*Make a note of how you feel.

Step 2 – Keeping eyes closed with head still

*Repeat the above step but with eyes closed.

Step 3 – Rotating head with eyes open

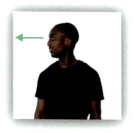 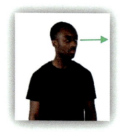

*Stand comfortably, keeping feet close together, facing forward.

*Rotate your head left and right for 20 seconds.

*Make a note of how you feel.

Step 4 – Rotating head with eyes closed

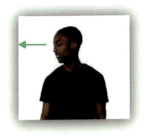 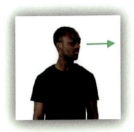

*Repeat the above step but with eyes closed.

Step 5 – Nodding head with eyes open

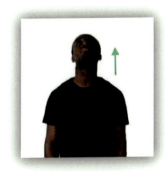

*Stand comfortably, keeping feet close together, facing forward.

*Nod head upwards and downwards for 20 seconds.

*Make a note of how you feel.

Step 6 – Nodding head with eyes closed

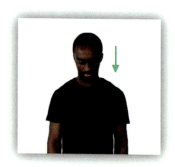

*Repeat the above step but with eyes closed.

Balance Test 4 – Difficulty: Hard

Tandem standing with various head movements

Step 1 – Keeping head still with eyes open

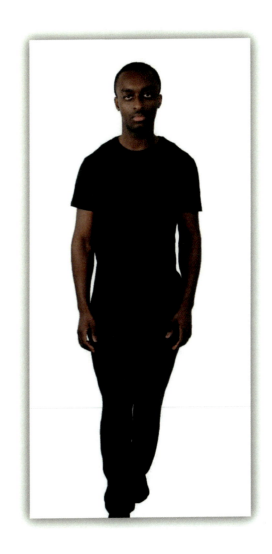

*Stand comfortably, keeping feet in a tandem position, facing forward.

*With eyes open, keep the body still for 20 seconds.

*Make a note of how you feel.

Step 2 – Keeping eyes closed with head still

*Repeat the above step but with eyes closed.

Step 3 – Rotating head with eyes open

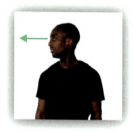 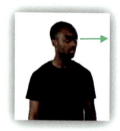

*Stand comfortably, keeping feet in a tandem position, facing forward.

*Rotate your head left and right for 20 seconds.

*Make a note of how you feel.

Step 4 – Rotating head with eyes closed

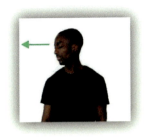 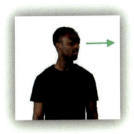

*Repeat the above step but with eyes closed.

Step 5 – Nodding head with eyes open

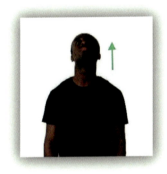

*Stand comfortably, keeping feet in a tandem position, facing forward.

*Nod head upwards and downwards for 20 seconds.

*Make a note of how you feel.

Step 6 – Nodding head with eyes closed

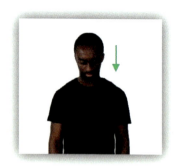

*Repeat the above step but with eyes closed.

Balance Test 5 – Difficulty: Hardest

Standing on one leg with various head movements

Step 1 – Keeping head still with eyes open

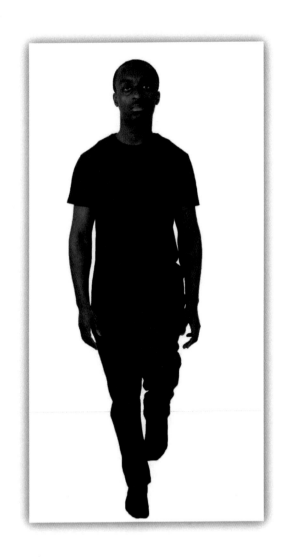

*Stand comfortably on one leg facing forward.

*With eyes open, keep the body still for 20 seconds.

*Make a note of how you feel.

Step 2 – Keeping eyes closed with head still

*Repeat the above step but with eyes closed.

Step 3 – Rotating head with eyes open

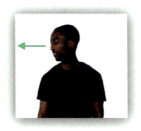 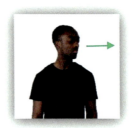

*Stand comfortably on one leg facing forward.

*Rotate your head left and right for 20 seconds.

*Make a note of how you feel.

Step 4 – Rotating head with eyes closed

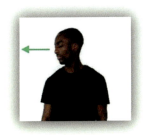 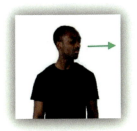

*Repeat the above step but with eyes closed.

Step 5 – Nodding head with eyes open

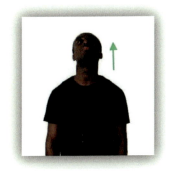

*Stand comfortably on one leg facing forward.

*Nod head upwards and downwards for 20 seconds.

*Make a note of how you feel.

Step 6 – Nodding head with eyes closed

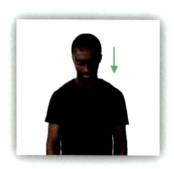

*Repeat the above step but with eyes closed.

Step 7 – Repeat steps 1-6 for the other leg.

> **Bonus Tip**
> You may notice that your balance feels different on the other leg. This is fine and you will improve your balance with both legs as you continue training.

Stage 6: Breakpoint Exercise: Abdominal Breathing

Performing the exercises within this guide can exert a lot of energy and can cause the body to build up stress and tension, especially when you're first starting out. So to prevent this from happening, we've incorporated some relaxation breakpoint exercises to bring your body to a calm state.

Once you've finished doing several repetitions of the exercises, it's time to begin the breakpoint exercise. Perform the following steps below:

1.) Sit comfortably on a chair, ensuring that your body is relaxed.

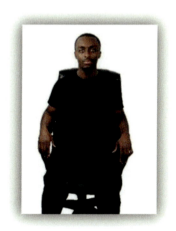

2.) Whilst keeping one hand on your stomach, slowly and quietly inhale through your nose for a count of 4 seconds. Your stomach should expand as you're doing this.

3.) Now hold your breath for two seconds.

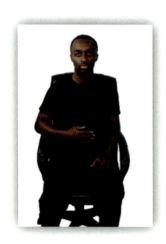

4.) Then, slowly and quietly exhale through your nose for a count of 4 seconds.

5.) Continue breathing like this for 1-2 minutes. You should feel much calmer and more relaxed once you've finished.

> **Bonus Tip**
> The key thing is to breathe from the abdomen and not the chest. Many people breathe in a shallow fashion, and practicing this exercise will help to correct your breathing pattern. This is also a good exercise to do throughout the day to further improve breathing.

Stage 7: Levels of Vestibular Progression

From beginner to expert, there are several levels that you can train at with these exercises. Below is a diagram that highlights each level, starting from the easiest level of training and progressing to the hardest.

Level of Progression for Body Positions/Movements

Easiest
- Lying down
- Sitting on chair
- Standing with feet wide apart
- Standing with feet in normal position
- Standing with feet close together
- Tandem standing with feet wide apart
- Tandem standing with feet close together
- Balancing on one leg
- Walking forward
- Walking backward

Hardest

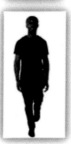

Level of Progression for Moving Head

Easiest
- Rotating Head
- Nodding Head

Hardest
- Moving Head Diagonally

Level of Progression for Moving Eyes

Easiest
- Eyes fixated straight
- Eyes moving at same time with head

Hardest
- Eyes moving in opposite direction to head

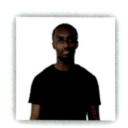

Standing Positions

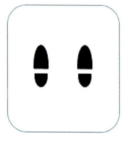

Normal foot position

Wide apart foot position

Narrow foot position

Wide tandem foot position

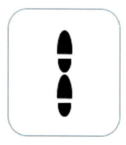

Close tandem foot position

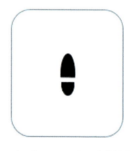

Balancing on one leg – left/right

The Vestibular Blueprint

Head movements + Eye Movements + Foot Position

This blueprint is extremely important to follow and is the key to training your vestibular system and balance.

Stage 8: The Exercises

Distant Gaze Stabilization

The first exercise that you will be doing is called Distant Gaze Stabilization.

1.) Select a body/standing position (e.g. sitting on a chair or standing in a normal foot position).

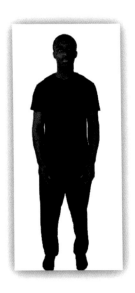

2.) Find a target or point to focus on in the distance (such as a cross on a wall). The target must be at around eye level.

3.) Rotate your head to the right while keeping your eyes fixated on the target. Make sure your eyes are always kept on the target.

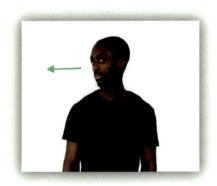

4.) Now rotate your head to the centre so that your head is facing forwards. Do not turn your head to the left as we only want your head to stop at the centre and not look towards your left.

5.) Do 2-4 repetitions of rotating your head to the right at a comfortable speed.

6.) Now perform 2-4 repetitions rotating your head to the left. Make sure that your head is stopping at the centre where your face is facing forwards.

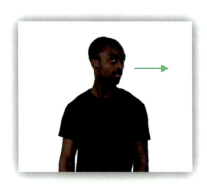

7.) Next, do 2-4 repetitions, this time moving your head upwards where your eyes are still focused on the target.

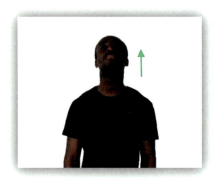

8.) Then do 2-4 repetitions nodding your head downwards, then going back to the centre.

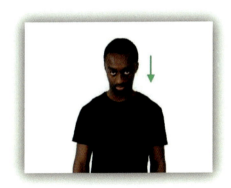

9.) Finally, do 2-4 repetitions moving your head in all 4 diagonal directions. These are usually the most difficult to do, so take your time with them. The directions are as follows:

*Head facing centre, then moving to the top left with eyes focused on the target.

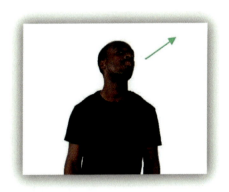

*Head facing centre, then moving to the bottom right with eyes focused on the target.

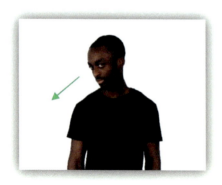

*Head facing centre, then moving to the top right with eyes focused on the target.

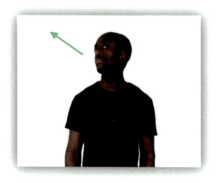

*Head facing centre, then moving to the bottom left with eyes focused on the target.

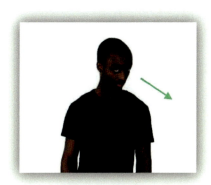

Bonus Tips

A.) When doing any of the exercises, you may have to start off really slow, where it may take you up to 1 MINUTE to do 1 repetition. This is normal. The important thing is to go at a pace that's comfortable for you, then gradually increase the speed that you do the exercises.

B.) You may notice that only 1 or 2 directions may not be functioning properly. In this case, you can focus on these areas first, then work on others.

C.) After each exercise, perform the Breakpoint exercise to prevent muscle tension from building up.

Close Range Gaze Stabilization

This exercise is known as Close Range Gaze Stabilization. It is similar to the Distant Gaze Stabilization exercise, but this time around you will be focusing on a point or target at a close range. This exercise is more challenging than the first exercise, where the closer the target you're focusing on is, the more challenging the exercise is to perform.

1.) Select a body/standing position (e.g. sitting on a chair or standing in a normal foot position).

> **Bonus Tip**
> There are 2 variations that this exercise can be performed in:
>
> A.) You can hold a pencil, pen or something similar in front of your face at eye level, at a distance that's around arm's length.
>
> B.) You can tape paper to a wall with a target on it (such as a cross "X") or something that you can focus your eyes on, ensuring that the target is at eye level and around arm's length.

2.) Once you've selected your variation, focus your eyes on the target and rotate your head to the right at a comfortable speed.

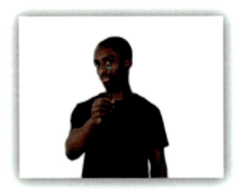

3.) Now rotate your head back to the centre. Make sure that you have only moved your head back just to the centre and not towards the left. Do 2-4 repetitions rotating your head to the right.

4.) Now perform 2-4 repetitions, rotating your head to the left and returning to the centre each time.

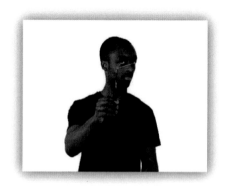

5.) Next, do 2-4 repetitions, starting with your head facing forwards, eyes focused on the target, moving your head upwards and returning to the centre.

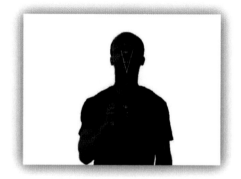

6.) After this, perform 2-4 repetitions with your head starting in the centre, moving your head downwards whilst your eyes are fixed on the target.

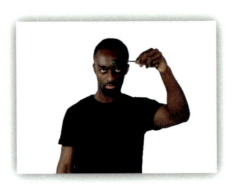

7.) Finally, do 2-4 repetitions, moving your head in all 4 diagonal directions. The directions are as follows:

*Head facing centre, then moving to the top left with eyes focused on the target.

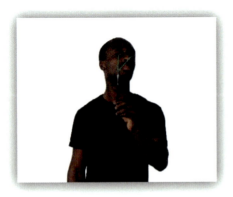

*Head facing centre, then moving to the bottom right with eyes focused on the target.

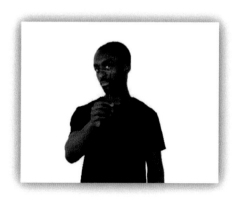

*Head facing centre, then moving to the top right with eyes focused on the target.

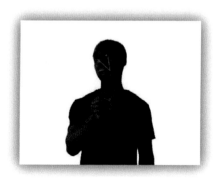

*Head facing centre, then moving to the bottom left with eyes focused on the target.

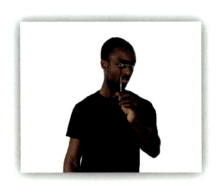

Joint Gaze Stabilization

This is exercise is called Joint Gaze Stabilization and is more challenging than the previous exercises. Instead of stopping at the centre at the end of each rep, we are now going to continue the movement onto the other side (e.g. moving our head from left to right). Ensure that you go at a comfortable pace when doing this exercise.

1.) Select a body/standing position (e.g. sitting on a chair or standing in a normal foot position).

Bonus Tip
There are 2 variations that this exercise can be performed in:

A.) You can hold a pencil, pen or something similar in front of your face at eye level, at a distance that's around arm's length.

B.) You can tape paper to a wall with a target on it (such as a cross "X") or something that you can focus your eyes on, ensuring that the target is at eye level and around arm's length.

2.) Rotate your head fully, moving from left to right whilst your eyes are fixated on the target. Do 2-4 repetitions of this at a comfortable pace.

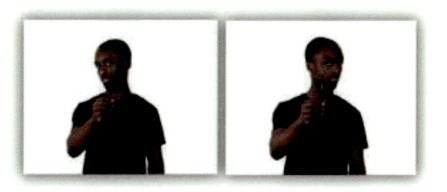

3.) Now fully nod your head upwards and downwards ensuring that you're moving your head as far possible, whilst still being able to clearly see the target. Perform 2-4 repetitions.

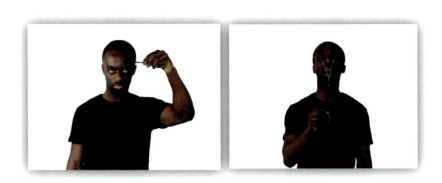

4.) Diagonally move your head towards the top left and bottom right with eyes on target. Do 2-4 repetitions.

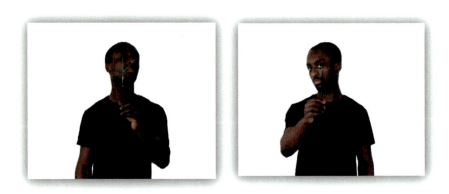

5.) Next, diagonally move your head towards the top right and bottom left with eyes on target. Do 2-4 repetitions.

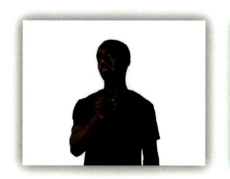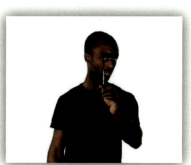

Combined Gaze Stabilization

Here we have our Combined Gaze Stabilization exercise. This is similar to the previous exercise, Joint Gaze Stabilization, but this time around instead of keeping your eyes fixed on one spot, your eyes and head will be moving at the same time.

1.) Select a body/standing position (e.g. sitting on a chair or standing in a normal foot position).

2.) With your left hand hold a pencil, pen or something similar in front of your face at eye level, at a distance that's around arm's length.

3.) Focusing your eyes on the target, move your left arm towards the left but at the same time also move your head towards the left as well. Your eyes and head should be in sync with each other. Ensure that you keep the rest of your body still.

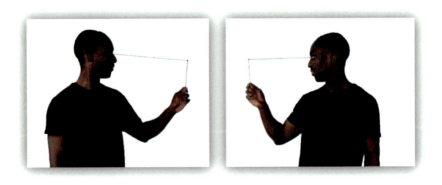

4.) Now move your left arm and head back towards the centre. As you reach the centre, switch arms and place your pen or target in your right hand and do the same as in Step 3 for your right side.

5.) Do 2-4 repetitions of these rotations using a comfortable speed.

6.) Now fully nod your head upwards and downwards ensuring that you're moving your head, eyes and pen or target together. Perform 2-4 repetitions.

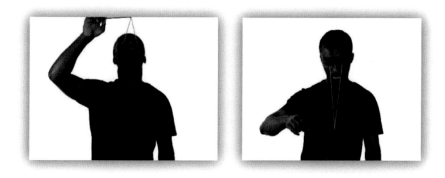

7.) Next, diagonally move your head towards the top left and bottom right with your eyes and pen or target together. Do 2-4 repetitions, switching hands at the centre of the head motion.

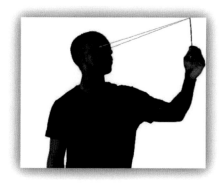
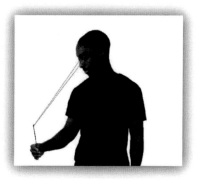

8.) Finally, diagonally move your head towards the top right and bottom left with your eyes and pen or target together. Do 2-4 repetitions, switching hands at the centre of the head motion.

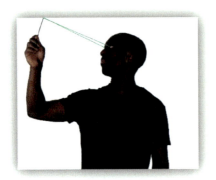 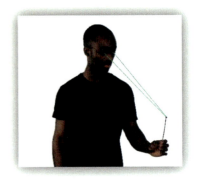

Rapid Gaze

This exercise is called Rapid Gaze. The type of eye movement we want to use for this exercise is called a saccade, which is being able to quickly move your eyes from one point to another. The goal of the exercise is to be able to quickly move your eyes to a target, and follow this up with a head movement. This skill is essential and is a movement that we perform on a regular basis. It will require you to use 2 targets.

1.) Select a body/standing position (e.g. sitting on a chair or standing in a normal foot position).

2.) Find 2 targets or pens to focus on, they should be about shoulder width apart from each other. The targets must be at around eye level at a distance that's around arm's length from yourself.

3.) Horizontally move your eyes towards the left as fast as you can, focusing on the first target. As soon as you can clearly see the target without any blurring, move your head towards the target so that your eyes and head are in-line with each other.

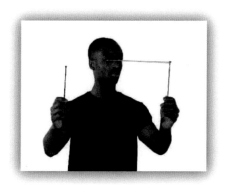

4.) With your head facing left, move your eyes towards the target on the right and once your vision is clear, move your head towards the right. Perform 2-4 repetitions going from left to right.

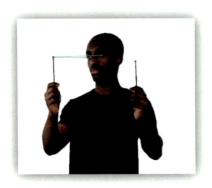

5.) Now rearrange your targets so that they are shoulder width apart but in a vertical manner. From here, with your head facing forwards move your eyes towards the target above, then follow that through with your head so that your head is facing the ceiling.

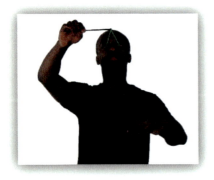

6.) From here, move your eyes to the target below, then follow through with your head – make sure your vision is clear before doing so. Perform 2-4 repetitions.

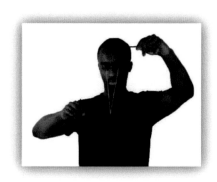

7.) It's now time for diagonals. Rearrange your targets so that one is in a top right location and the other is in a bottom left location. Whilst you're facing the centre, move your eyes towards the target located at the top right, then follow through with your head.

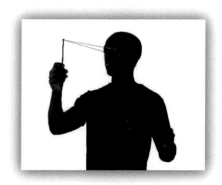

8.) From here, move your eyes towards the bottom left, then move your head. Perform 2-4 repetitions.

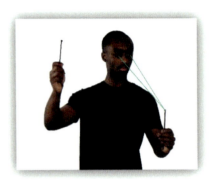

9.) Finally, rearrange your targets so that one is in a top left location and the other is in a bottom right location. Whilst facing forwards, move your eyes towards the target located at the top left, then follow through with your head.

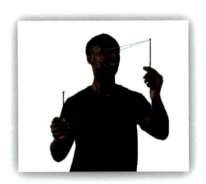

10.) From here, move your eyes towards the bottom right, then move your head. Perform 2-4 repetitions.

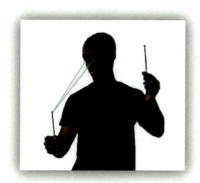

Bonus Tip
As you improve with this exercise, your aim is to be able to move your eyes, then your head as quickly as possible. This ability will develop as you continue to practice this exercise.

Opposing Gaze

This next exercise is known as opposing gaze. It is one of the most challenging exercises in this guide. The way this exercise works is by moving your head in one direction, whilst your target (e.g. your pen) and your eyes are moving in the opposing direction. When you first start practicing this exercise, start off with a small range of motion (distance) and only focus in one area or direction (similar to how the Close Range Gaze Stabilization exercise was performed, where you worked in 8 separate directions).

1.) Select a body/standing position (e.g. sitting on a chair or standing in a normal foot position).

2.) With your left hand, hold a pencil, pen or something similar in front of your face at eye level, at a distance that's around arm's length.

3.) Focusing your eyes on the target, rotate your head towards the right whilst moving your left arm and eyes towards the left.

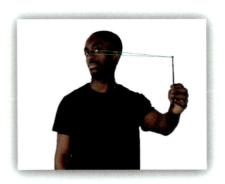

4.) Now move your left arm and head back towards the centre. Repeat Step 3 again and perform 2-4 repetitions at a comfortable speed.

5.) Next, place your pen or target in your right hand and do the same action, performing 2-4 repetitions. Ensure that you rotate your head towards the left whilst moving your eyes and arm towards the right.

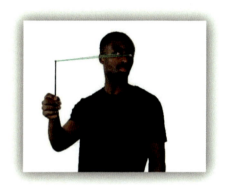

6.) Then move your head downwards whilst moving your eyes and target upwards. Do 2-4 repetitions, bringing your head and arm back to the centre at the end of each repetition.

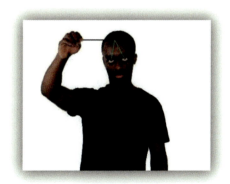

7.) After this, move your head upwards whilst moving your eyes and target downwards. Do 2-4 repetitions whilst bringing your head and arm back to the centre at the end of each repetition.

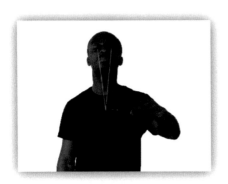

8.) For the diagonal directions perform 2-4 repetitions doing the following:

*Head rotating towards the top left with eyes and target moving towards the bottom right.

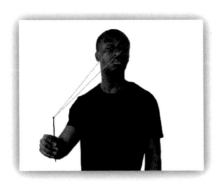

*Head rotating towards the bottom right with eyes and target moving towards the top left.

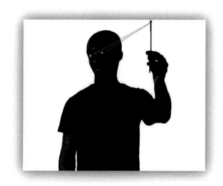

*Head rotating towards the top right with eyes and target moving towards the bottom left.

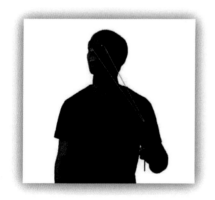

*Head rotating towards the bottom left with eyes and target moving towards the top right.

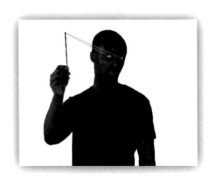

Body Swaying

For the Body Swaying exercise, the goal is to integrate (put together) all 3 sensory systems where they can all work in sync with each other. This exercise may seem simple to do at first, but can be very challenging as you perform more repetitions.

1.) Select a body/standing position (e.g. sitting on a chair or standing in a normal foot position).

2.) Keep your entire body as still and upright as possible. It may help to visualise yourself in a straight and upright position.

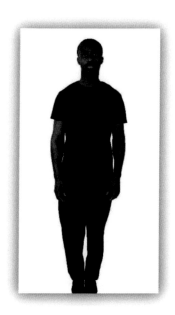

3.) Find a target or point to focus on in the distance (such as a cross on a wall). The target must be at around eye level.

4.) Begin swaying your entire body forwards and backwards, whilst keeping your eyes fixed on your target. Do 2-4 repetitions.

5.) Remember to keep your body as still as possible – no bending of any body parts such as the back or knees. Visualise yourself upright if this helps.

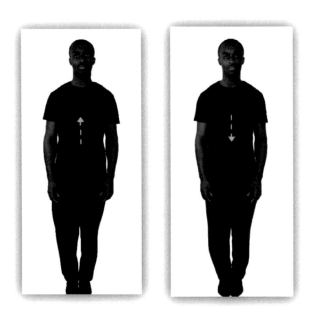

6.) Next, start swaying your body left to right. You don't have to add a lot of motion with this, just enough so that you can feel yourself swaying. Do 2-4 repetitions.

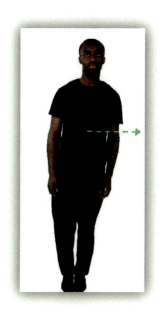 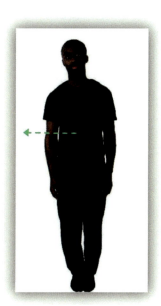

7.) Now you will sway diagonally.

*Begin swaying forwards-right, then backwards-left. Do 2-4 repetitions.

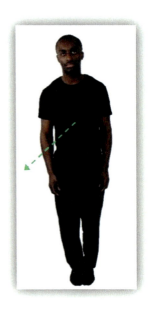 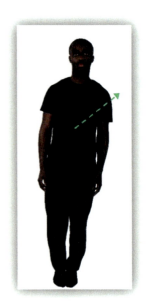

*Begin swaying forwards-left, then backwards-right. Do 2-4 repetitions.

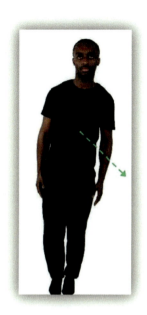 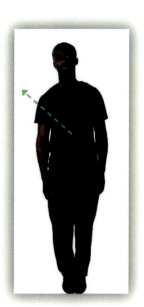

8.) Finally, move your entire body in circles whilst facing forwards, clockwise and counter-clockwise. Do 2-4 repetitions in both directions.

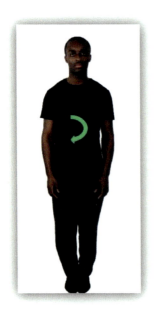 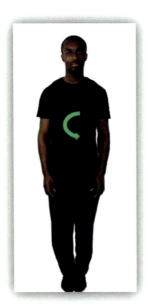

Walking With Head Movements

Standard Gaze Variation – Easier Version

The last exercise is another integration exercise. This exercise will incorporate the majority of the previous exercises that you have done so far. Pay close attention as this is a vital exercise.

1.) Find a location where you will be able to walk a minimum of 5-8 steps. Narrow passages/hallways are great for this exercise, as in the event that you lose your balance, you can grab on to a wall.

2.) Focus on a target that is directly in front of you at around eye level.

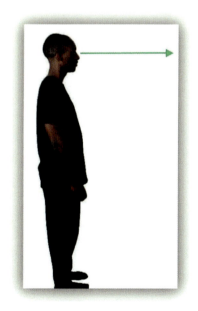

3.) Start off by walking forward, as slowly and as comfortably as possible. As you're doing this, rotate your head left and right and stop after you've walked 5-8 steps.

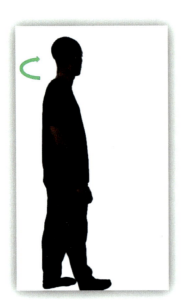 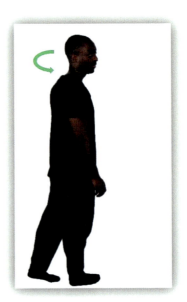

4.) Turn around and focus your eyes on a target at around eye level, then walk forward for about 5-8 steps whilst rotating your head.

Bonus Tip
Once you are comfortable performing this exercise, instead of turning around you can do the same exercise but walking backwards. This is an advanced variation and should only be done once you're comfortable doing the exercise walking forward.

5.) This time, perform the same exercise again but instead of rotating your head whilst walking forward, nod your head upwards and downwards whilst keeping your eyes on the target.

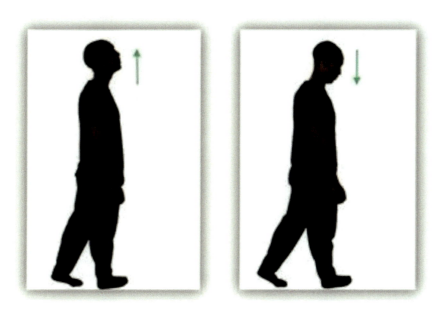

6.) Finally, do the same again but this time around, rotate your head diagonally – make sure to do both directions (top left to bottom right and top right to bottom left).

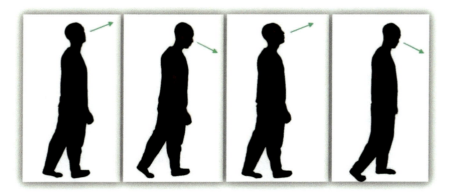

Walking With Head Movements

Combined Gaze Variation – Challenging Version

1.) Find a location where you will be able to walk a minimum of 5-8 steps. Narrow passages/hallways are great for this exercise, as in the event that you lose your balance, you can grab on to a wall.

2.) Start off by walking forward, as slowly and as comfortably as possible.

As you're doing so, rotate your head and eyes left and right – your eyes and head should be moving together and in sync with each other. You should NOT be focusing your eyes on a target with this exercise. Stop after you've walked 5-8 steps.

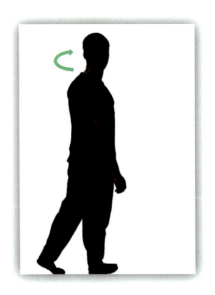 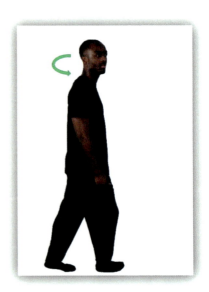

3.) Turn around and perform Step 2 again, stopping after 5-8 steps.

4.) This time, perform the same exercise again but instead of rotating your head and eyes together whilst walking forward, nod your head upwards and downwards whilst keeping your eyes and head in sync together.

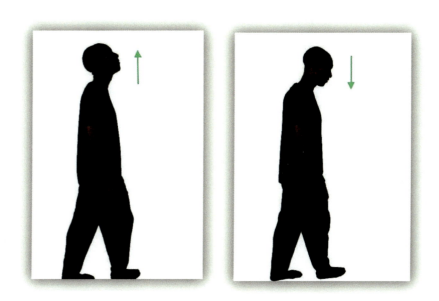

5.) Finally do the same again but this time around rotate your head diagonally whilst keeping your eyes and head in sync together. Make sure to do both directions (top left to bottom right and top right to bottom left).

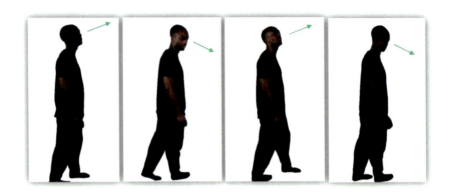

Bonus Tip
Once you are comfortable performing this exercise, instead of turning around you can do the same exercise but walking backwards. This is an advanced variation and should only be done once you're comfortable doing the exercise walking forward.

Stage 9: What Next?

The Vertigo Treatment Course - Your Reward!

As our way of saying thank you for investing into The Vertigo Treatment guide, we wanted to reward you with an 88% discount off The Vertigo Treatment course. This course is a simple, step-by-step video tutorial course, that goes over the exercises and drills in more detail. In addition, you will have access to one-on-one support, where any questions you may have can be answered. There are also many bonus exercises and drills available, which aren't present within this guide.

This is perfect for those who want to gain more clarity and understanding on how to perform the exercises and drills, for those who want to speed up their recovery from vertigo and for those who want access to additional one-on-one support.

Enrol now: http://www.curevertigonow.com/get-started

*Those who enrol will save 88% off the original price. This special offer will be available for a limited time only.

Join Our Support Group

If you're in need of any support, feel free to join our support group. We are always here to help:

https://www.facebook.com/groups/curevertigonow

Connect With Us

Website: http://www.curevertigonow.com

Facebook: https://www.facebook.com/curevertigonow

Twitter: https://twitter.com/curevertigonow

YouTube:
https://www.youtube.com/channel/UCYbbNQf_Z2OkYvuzzYiXeEg

We look forward to seeing your results and remember to keep on propelling forward!

Made in the USA
Middletown, DE
03 February 2021